DEBORAH LYNNE BOYD

The Menopause Handbook
A Simple Guide For The Moden Woman

To the sisterhood of women everywhere,
This book is dedicated to you – the brave, the resilient, the nurturers
and the warriors.
You are not alone on this journey. Your experiences are valid, your
feelings are important, and your health matters.

Contents

One

Introduction

Welcome to 'The Menopause Handbook,' a comprehensive easy to understand guide designed to demystify the various stages of menopause so you can navigate your way through the transition of menopause with more understanding and confidence.

I wrote this book due to my own experiences of menopause and the challenges I faced trying to understand what was happening to me and then to get the support I needed.

I was persistently curious and sought out help from several doctors and found that many of them were not willing to talk about menopause and some were completely opposed to any type of treatment.

As my own journey of discovery unfolded, I found that women

and men were poorly informed about menopause and many women had no idea about current treatment options (me included) so I decided to learn for myself and then share the information.

This book is structured to provide you with a clear understanding of what to expect during menopause, addressing common symptoms such as hot flashes, sleep disturbances, mood swings and many more. You will learn about the hormonal changes that underpin these experiences, offering simple explanations for the changes occurring within your body.

Each section of the book is designed to equip you with knowledge and will hopefully, answer some of your questions. 'The Menopause Handbook' is a simple, straightforward, guide for navigating the physical and emotional complexities of menopause so you understand how to preserve your well-being and maintain your quality of life.

I hope it helps answer some of your questions and gives you the courage to start your own journey to find solutions that help and support you. The bottom line is that you do have choices.

Two

Disclaimer

This book is primarily focused on the experience of menopause as it relates to individuals who were assigned female at birth and identify as women. The information and discussions herein are based on this demographic due to the biological and physiological aspects of menopause typically associated with female reproductive health.

I acknowledge and respect the diversity of gender identities and experiences. This book does not intend to overlook or diminish the experiences of individuals who, despite not identifying as women, may also undergo menopausal changes due to various medical, hormonal, or surgical reasons.

The content of this book should not be taken as comprehensive or exclusive of all menopausal experiences. It is not intended to be exclusionary or to invalidate the experiences of gender-diverse individuals who may be affected by menopause.

My aim is to provide information and support to those experiencing menopause, understanding that this can encompass a wide range of individuals with diverse gender identities.

Readers are encouraged to seek information and resources that are inclusive of their personal experiences and identities. I advocate for the recognition and understanding of menopause as a human experience, beyond the confines of gender labels, and I support all individuals on their unique journeys through this life stage.

Three

Menopause Overview

Stages

Menopause is defined by three stages:

Peri-menopause – This is described as the transition into menopause. **The period in a woman's life when she starts to experience hormonal fluctuations and changes to her periods.** The average time for a woman to be peri-menopausal is between four and five years. During this time, periods may change and become shorter or longer and many other menopause symptoms can be experienced. Peri-menopause typically starts in your 40's but can start in your 30's.

Menopause – This marks the end of a woman's menstrual cycle and is usually diagnosed when you have gone 12 months without a period. It can occur in your 40's – 50's or even earlier and surgical menopause can occur if you have to have your ovaries removed surgically for some reason.

Post-menopause – The period after menopause has occurred, this starts when you have not had a period for 12 months.

A point to note is that it can be tricky to fully understand the stage you are in if you have had a hysterectomy (removal of your uterus) and don't have periods to monitor.

Menopause Symptoms

The symptoms of menopause are many and varied and can occur in isolation or several together all at once. Irregular periods are often one of the first signs of menopause, and these signal changes in the reproductive system as it transitions away from fertility. Each woman's experience with symptoms is unique, and what happens to one may not happen to another. It may take some trial and error to find the most effective management strategies that work for you.

My journey started with night sweats, I was waking up every night drenched and not sure why. Having to get up and change pyjamas disrupted my sleep, making work really challenging the next day. I remember discussing it with my doctor and he did a blood test and confirmed I was "peri-menopausal" and that night sweats were part of the deal, but didn't offer any suggestions of how to cope with them. I was busy working full time, parenting teenage boys with my hubby and didn't really have time for me, so just struggled on.

Hot flashes and night sweats are some of the most frequently reported symptoms. Less commonly known symptoms are joint pain, which can make you worry you have developed arthritis. Brain fog, affecting your memory and concentration that can interfere with your work. Mood swings and rapid changes in emotion can make you wonder what on earth is happening to you and you end up losing your confidence.

There are several other symptoms which are rarely talked about but are equally important, symptoms like vaginal dryness, which can cause discomfort and affect your desire for sex, along with various bladder symptoms such as increased frequency or urgency of urination (you know that feeling when you just have to pee!!).

The following chapters will provide more detailed information, and offer suggestions for management and treatment options. The goal is to provide a thorough understanding of these symptoms, enabling you to identify and understand each one and consider your treatment options to effectively maintain your comfort and quality of life.

Below are some common definitions of symptoms:

Hot Flashes: A common symptom characterized by sudden, intense heat spreading through the upper body, often accompanied by sweating and a reddened face. They can vary in frequency and intensity and may be triggered by various factors, including spicy food, caffeine, and stress.

Night Sweats: These are severe hot flashes that occur at night and can disrupt sleep. They may cause excessive perspiration, leading to discomfort and sleep disturbances that can impact daily functioning.

Joint Pain: Menopausal women often report increased joint pain, which may be linked to hormonal changes. This pain can affect any joint but is commonly felt in the hips, knees, and hands.

Brain Fog: A term used to describe cognitive impairments during menopause, including difficulties with memory, focus, and the ability to perform mental tasks. It is often transient and can be managed through lifestyle adjustments.

Mood Swings: Emotional volatility (ups and downs) is another symptom attributed to the hormonal fluctuations of menopause. Women may experience sudden changes in mood, such as feeling irritable, anxious, or depressed.

Sleep Disturbances: The quality of sleep can be significantly affected during menopause, with issues like insomnia, waking up frequently during the night, and not feeling rested after sleep.

Vaginal Dryness: Decreased oestrogen levels can lead to reduced natural lubrication, causing discomfort, itching, or pain, particularly during sex.

Bladder Symptoms: Menopause can lead to urinary issues such as increased urgency, frequent peeing, and an increased risk of urinary tract infections.

Weight Gain: This is common during menopause due to hormonal changes, metabolic slow down, loss of muscle mass and sleep disturbance.

Irregular Periods: As a woman approaches menopause, her periods may become irregular. Periods may be shorter or longer, lighter or heavier, or have a more erratic schedule before ceasing entirely.

Four

Hormonal Changes

In this chapter, we delve into the hormonal shifts that are at the heart of the menopause transition. Understanding oestrogen's wide-ranging effects can be crucial for managing menopause symptoms effectively.

Oestrogen in particular affects many of the body's systems and there are a variety of strategies available to minimise the effects of its decline during menopause. These strategies encompass lifestyle modifications, nutritional supplementation, and, if required, medical treatments. It is really important that you understand the changes that are happening and are informed and able to seek help and support when you need it.

Decline in Oestrogen and Progesterone Levels

The decline in oestrogen and progesterone levels is central

to most of the physical and emotional symptoms women experience during this time.

Oestrogen and progesterone are the primary female reproductive hormones produced by the ovaries. As menopause approaches, the ovaries gradually produce less of these hormones resulting in various symptoms which include night sweats, joint aches, hot flashes and brain fog (to name a few) and eventually there is a decrease in your periods cycle regularity and your periods finally stop.

This reduction in hormone levels can lead to various symptoms discussed in the previous chapter and have long-term effects on other systems in the body.

Cardiovascular System: Oestrogen plays a protective role in heart health by maintaining the flexibility of the arteries, allowing them to accommodate blood flow easily. It also helps regulate cholesterol levels, promoting the balance between good (HDL) and bad (LDL) cholesterol. The decline in oestrogen during menopause can therefore increase your risk of developing cardiovascular diseases.

Skeletal System: Oestrogen is crucial for bone health; it helps to balance the process of bone remodelling by preventing excessive bone resorption, which is when bone tissue is broken down to release minerals into the blood. Lower oestrogen levels can lead to an acceleration of bone loss, increasing the risk of osteoporosis.

Brain Function: Oestrogen has several neuroprotective roles.

It can enhance neuronal growth and the formation of neural connections. It is also thought to have a beneficial effect on neurotransmitter systems that influence mood, cognitive function, and memory. As oestrogen levels drop, some women may experience mood swings, memory lapses, and a decrease in cognitive function (you forget stuff).

Metabolic Impact: Oestrogen affects body weight and composition. It influences fat distribution, metabolism, and insulin sensitivity. With the reduction of oestrogen, women often experience changes in body fat distribution, increased abdominal fat, and sometimes an increased risk of metabolic syndrome and type 2 diabetes.

Urinary Tract: Oestrogen helps to keep the tissues of the urinary tract elastic. A decrease in oestrogen levels can lead to the weakening of the urinary tract tissues, contributing to incontinence or increased urinary tract infections.

Skin and Hair: Oestrogen contributes to skin elasticity and moisture by increasing collagen production and skin thickness. It also affects hair growth. As oestrogen levels decline, women may notice their skin becomes drier and less elastic, and hair may become thinner or fall out more easily.

Impact on the Endocrine System

The endocrine system, responsible for hormone production and regulation, experiences significant changes as oestrogen and progesterone levels decline. These changes can disrupt the delicate balance of the body's endocrine functions, affecting not just the reproductive system but also influencing metabolism, mood regulation, and thermal regulation, which is why hot flashes and night sweats occur.

The endocrine system's response to menopause is complex and interconnected. The changes can be subtle or more pronounced, affecting not just reproductive health but overall well-being. Understanding these processes is essential for managing symptoms effectively and maintaining health during and after the menopause transition.

Five

Managing Hot Flashes

Managing hot flashes is a priority for many women during menopause, as this is one of the most common and often most uncomfortable symptoms.

Lifestyle Changes

- Dress in Layers: This allows for quick adjustments to changes in body temperature.
- Stay Cool: Use fans, cooling sprays, or moist wipes. At night, use light bedding and breathable cotton pyjamas.
- Mind Your Diet: Spicy foods, caffeine, and alcohol can trigger hot flashes in some women.
- Quit Smoking: Smoking is linked to increased hot flashes.

Dietary Adjustments you can make

- Soy Products: Include more foods high in phytoestrogens, like soy for example, it may offer some relief from hot flashes.
- Stay Hydrated: Drink plenty of water to help regulate body temperature.

Supplements and Herbal Remedies: Some women find relief in herbal remedies but there is no research to support their effectiveness. Their use should always be discussed with your healthcare provider as some herbal remedies can have negative interactions with medications.

- Vitamin E: Some women find relief from hot flashes with vitamin E supplements.
- Black Cohosh: A commonly used herb that may reduce hot flashes,

Medical Treatments

- Hormone Replacement Therapy (HRT): This is considered the most effective treatment for most menopause symptoms including hot flashes but it's not suitable for everyone. It's important to discuss the benefits and risks associated with HRT with your doctor so you are fully informed before you start using it.
- Prescription Medications: Certain antidepressants, anticonvulsants, and blood pressure medications have been found to be effective for some women. These too should be

discussed with your doctor so you fully understand your options.

Alternative Therapies

- Acupuncture: Some studies suggest acupuncture can help reduce the frequency and severity of hot flashes.
- Yoga and Exercise: Regular physical activity may help reduce hot flashes and improve sleep quality.

Six

Managing Night Sweats and Sleep Disturbances

When I started having night sweats I wondered what on earth was going on and had no clue they might be due to menopause. For some reason, I just didn't connect them together. As I discovered they can be very disruptive and managing them can be tricky and require lots of trial and error, ultimately you are trying to preserve your sleep quality so you can still function through the day.

You can make choices about your bedroom environment and your bedtime routines, but it's important to note that while these strategies can be helpful, they may not completely eliminate night sweats. Maintaining a sleep diary to track triggers and patterns can provide useful insights and help you and your healthcare provider create a more effective management plan. Some of the following options might work for you.

Bedroom Environment

- **Cool Temperature:** Keep the bedroom at a cool, comfortable temperature and use a fan or air conditioning if necessary.
- **Breathable Bedding:** Use sheets and blankets made of natural, breathable fibres like cotton.
- **Layered Clothing:** Wear lightweight, loose-fitting pyjamas made from natural fibres to allow for easy adjustment as your body temperature changes.

Sleep Hygiene: It's important to practice good sleep hygiene, such as maintaining a regular sleep schedule and creating a comfortable, sleep-conducive environment in the bedroom. Read a book prior to sleeping and stay off your devices limiting your exposure to blue light.

You may need to alter your daily routine for a while so speak with your employer and see if you can rearrange your start and finish times.

Lifestyle Modifications

- Hydration: Drink cool water throughout the day and keep a glass by your bed at night.
- Avoid Triggers: Steer clear of spicy foods, caffeine, and alcohol close to bedtime, as they can trigger night sweats.
- Regular Exercise: Engaging in regular physical activity

during the day can improve overall body temperature regulation.

Stress Management

- Relaxation Techniques: Activities such as reading, gentle yoga, or meditation before bed can help reduce stress, which in turn can help lessen the severity of night sweats.
- Breathing techniques: Being woken by a night sweat can make you feel really frustrated and deep, slow abdominal breathing exercises can help to calm you down, making it easier to fall back asleep.

Dietary Adjustments:

- Avoid Heavy Meals Before Bed: A light, easily digestible snack is better than a large meal that can increase your body's metabolic rate and internal temperature. I try to stop eating around 7.30 PM.

Medical Treatments

- Hormone Replacement Therapy (HRT): This is considered the most effective treatment for most menopause symptoms including night sweats, but it's not suitable for everyone. It's important to discuss the benefits and risks associated with HRT so you are fully informed before you

start using it.
- Prescription Medications: Certain non-hormonal medications, like antidepressants and anticonvulsants, can reduce the frequency of night sweats for some women. These too should be discussed with your doctor so you fully understand your options.

Alternative Therapies

- Herbal Supplements: Some women find relief with herbs such as black cohosh, but their efficacy and safety should be discussed with a healthcare provider.
- Acupuncture: This traditional Chinese medicine technique may help some women manage their symptoms.
- Yoga and Exercise: Regular physical activity may help improve sleep quality.

Seven

Managing Joint Pain and Bone Health

In this chapter, we focus on how to manage joint pain and the critical issue of bone health during and post-menopause, a period marked by increased vulnerability to osteoporosis due to hormonal changes. I experienced terrible pain in the joints in my hands and thought I was developing arthritis. Investigations by a Rheumatologist advised my hands were normal but no one mentioned menopause as a possible cause. I have since discovered it's not an uncommon symptom but no one tells you this.

Managing Joint Pain

Joint pain is a common complaint during menopause, which may be associated with the broader changes affecting bone health. Pain is more commonly experienced in hips, knees and hands. Strategies for managing joint pain, include lifestyle modifications, medical treatments, and complementary therapies.

Non-pharmacological Interventions: These include lifestyle modifications such as regular exercise tailored to reduce stress on the joints, like swimming or cycling, which can improve joint flexibility and strength without excessive impact. Weight management is also crucial, as excess body weight can increase stress on weight-bearing joints.

Heat and Cold Therapy: Applying heat can relax muscles and increase blood flow for relief of joint stiffness, while cold therapy can reduce inflammation and numb the areas experiencing acute pain.

Physical Therapy: A physical therapist can develop a personalized exercise program that includes specific stretches and strengthening exercises to help maintain joint function and alleviate pain.

Nutritional Supplements: Certain supplements, such as glucosamine and chondroitin, omega-3 fatty acids, and curcumin, have been suggested to help reduce joint pain and inflammation. Clinical studies have had mixed results however and their effectiveness is not guaranteed.

Medications: Over-the-counter pain relievers such as NSAIDs (e.g., ibuprofen) may be used for pain management, but long-term use should be monitored due to potential side effects. In some cases, prescription medications may be necessary, and a doctor can provide the best guidance on these.

Alternative Therapies: Acupuncture and massage therapy are popular alternatives that some find helpful for managing joint pain.

Hormone Replacement Therapy (HRT): For some women, HRT can alleviate joint pain by stabilizing hormone levels, though the risks and benefits should be thoroughly discussed with a healthcare provider.

Osteoporosis Risk During and After Menopause

The risk of osteoporosis significantly escalates during and after menopause due to the steep decline in oestrogen levels. Women can lose up to 20% of their bone density in the five to seven years following menopause, which substantially increases the risk of osteoporosis. This condition is often referred to as a "silent disease" because it can progress without any symptoms until a fracture occurs. Fractures related to osteoporosis are more common in the hip, spine, and wrist, and such injuries can have significant long-term impacts on your mobility and independence.

Risk factors for osteoporosis include a family history of the disease, a small body frame, a history of fractures, certain medical conditions and medications, smoking, and excessive alcohol consumption. Ethnicity also plays a role, with Caucasian and Asian women at higher risk.

Bone density tests, also known as DEXA scans, are recommended for all women aged 65 and older and for younger women with a heightened risk of fractures. These tests can detect osteoporosis before a fracture occurs and can also monitor bone density over time.

Preventive strategies are crucial and include ensuring adequate intake of calcium and vitamin D, engaging in regular weight-bearing and muscle-strengthening exercises, avoiding smoking and excessive alcohol, and considering medication when appropriate.

Importance of Calcium and Vitamin D

Calcium and vitamin D are essential for maintaining bone health. Calcium is the primary mineral found in bones, and vitamin D is necessary for calcium absorption and bone growth.

Calcium is the cornerstone of bone health. Women are generally recommended to consume between 1,000 mg to 1,200 mg of calcium daily, with the higher intake often suggested for those in postmenopausal states. Dietary sources of calcium include dairy products like milk, cheese, and yogurt; leafy green vegetables; nuts; and calcium-fortified foods like certain cereals and plant-based milk.

Vitamin D plays an equally important role because it facilitates the absorption of calcium from the gut into the bloodstream. Without sufficient vitamin D, the body cannot absorb calcium effectively, regardless of how much is consumed. Vitamin D is also involved in bone remodelling and repair. It can be obtained from exposure to sunlight, which triggers its production in the skin, as well as from dietary sources such as fatty fish, liver, egg yolks, and fortified foods.

The recommended daily allowance for vitamin D is more challenging to specify due to individual variations in sunlight exposure and dietary intake, but many experts suggest at least 600 to 800 IU per day, with higher doses often recommended for older adults.

Exercise and Bone Density

Exercise is also important for osteoporosis prevention and management, playing a significant role in maintaining and improving bone density, particularly during and after menopause. Physical activity, especially weight-bearing and resistance exercises, is shown to stimulate bone formation and slow the loss of bone density.

Weight-bearing Exercises

These are activities that make you move against gravity while staying upright. They force your body to work against gravity and stimulate bone cells to grow. Weight-bearing exercises include walking, hiking, jogging, climbing stairs, playing tennis, and dancing.

Resistance Training

This type of exercise involves the use of weights or resistance bands to build muscle mass and bone strength. Resistance training can include activities such as lifting weights, using resistance bands, and doing body-weight exercises like push-ups and squats. The benefits of these exercises for bone health are twofold: they not only increase bone density but also improve balance, coordination, and muscle strength, all of which can help prevent falls and related fractures.

Frequency and Intensity

For maximum bone health benefits, it's recommended that adults engage in at least 30 minutes of moderate-intensity weight-bearing exercise on most days of the week. Resistance training should be done 2 to 3 times per week, targeting all the major muscle groups.

Tailored Exercise Programs

Please remember to consult with your healthcare professional before starting any new exercise programme to ensure they tailor your exercise regimen to your fitness level and bone health status. For those already diagnosed with osteoporosis, some high-impact exercises may not be safe due to the increased risk of fracture. In such cases, low-impact exercises, such as brisk walking or elliptical training, can be effective.

Eight

Managing Brain Fog and Memory Lapses and Cognitive Function

This chapter focuses on managing brain fog and memory lapses that can occur during menopause and provides strategies to maintain and support brain health. The easiest example I can give is when you have something to say (it's on the tip of your tongue) and you just lose it, the words just don't come. It's both frustrating and embarrassing. It's really important to prioritise your own personal well-being if you experience these symptoms. There are several strategies to follow that may help.

Cognitive Changes During Menopause

Many women experience symptoms such as brain fog, memory lapses, difficulty concentrating, and problems with executive function (the thinking processes that help us get things done).

These cognitive symptoms are often transient and are thought to be related to the fluctuating levels of hormones, particularly oestrogen, which has a protective effect on the brain and is involved in the neurotransmitter function and cognitive processes.

Brain Health and Strategies to Maintain Cognitive Function

Keeping your brain functioning and maintaining brain health during menopause involves a combination of lifestyle habits, mental exercises, and possibly medical interventions:

- **Mental Stimulation:** Engaging in activities that challenge the brain, such as puzzles, learning new skills, or taking educational courses, can help keep the mind sharp. Learning new skills or new information has a very positive effect on brain function
- **Physical Exercise:** Regular physical activity increases blood flow to the brain and can improve cognitive functions. It also helps in reducing the risk of diseases that can impair cognitive health, such as cardiovascular disease.
- **Nutrition:** A diet rich in antioxidants, omega-3 fatty acids, and other brain-healthy nutrients can support cognitive function. Foods such as leafy greens, berries, nuts, and fish are particularly beneficial.
- **Sleep Quality:** Good sleep is essential for cognitive health. Sleep disturbances should be addressed, as they can significantly impact memory and concentration. Re-establishing sleep habits can have a really positive impact on your well-being. When you sleep better you function

better.

- **Stress Management:** Chronic stress can impair cognitive function. Stress-reducing practices like meditation, yoga, and deep breathing can be beneficial.
- **Social Engagement:** Maintaining social connections and engaging in regular social activities can support cognitive health and emotional well-being.
- **Health Check-Ups:** Regular check-ups can help manage health conditions that might affect cognitive health, such as hypertension or diabetes.
- **Hormone Replacement Therapy (HRT):** This may help manage menopausal symptoms, including cognitive changes, it should be discussed with your healthcare provider and considered along with other solutions

Nine

Managing Mood Swings – Psychological And Emotional Wellbeing

In this chapter, we turn our attention to the psychological and emotional landscape of menopause, an area that can significantly influence a woman's experience of this life stage.

It can feel like a really lonely time where you are losing yourself. Understanding what is happening in your body can really help to navigate the process and being able to speak about how you are feeling and what is happening for you as an individual, is really important for supporting your mental health and emotional resilience. The value of the sisterhood is real.

Menopausal Mood Changes: Hormonal fluctuations during

menopause can lead to mood swings characterised by emotional highs and lows. You may find yourself feeling irritable or experiencing sudden bouts of sadness or happiness without a clear cause.

These mood swings are common and can be a very distressing symptom. They are characterized by rapid fluctuations in mood, which can range from joy to sadness or irritability without a clear trigger. These mood swings can be attributed to the hormonal changes that occur during menopause, primarily the fluctuations in oestrogen levels. Oestrogen interacts with chemicals in the brain that affect mood, including serotonin and endorphins. Besides the direct biochemical effects, the physical symptoms of menopause, such as sleep disturbances and hot flashes, can also exacerbate mood swings due to fatigue and stress.

The management of menopausal mood swings often includes a combination of lifestyle interventions, psychological strategies, and medical treatments. Lifestyle modifications such as regular exercise, adequate sleep, a balanced diet, and stress reduction techniques can help to stabilize your mood. Psychological strategies may involve cognitive-behavioural therapy or other forms of counselling to develop coping skills. In some cases, hormone replacement therapy (HRT) or other medications, like antidepressants, may be recommended to help regulate mood swings, but these should always be considered in consultation with a healthcare provider due to potential risks and side effects.

Loss of Confidence: The period of menopause often coincides with significant life events or transitions, such as children leaving home (the "empty nest" syndrome), caring for ageing parents, weight gain or dealing with personal health concerns, which can contribute to feelings of sadness, loss, or anxiety. These challenging situations can also lead to a decrease in self-esteem and confidence.

Anxiety and Depression: Menopause can be a trigger for anxiety and depression in some women. The changes in hormone levels, combined with the stresses of middle age, can contribute to the onset or exacerbation of these conditions.

Anxiety: Many women may experience heightened anxiety during menopause, which can manifest as general feelings of nervousness, panic attacks, or obsessive-compulsive behaviours. Fluctuations in oestrogen and progesterone can affect neurotransmitter systems in the brain that regulate mood, potentially leading to increased anxiety. Additionally, other menopausal symptoms like hot flashes and sleep disturbances can exacerbate anxiety symptoms.

Depression: The risk of depression may increase during menopause. While the drop in hormone levels is a factor, the psychological impact of physical changes such as weight gain, ageing, and decreased fertility can also play a role. Depression during menopause is not just about mood; it can affect energy levels, appetite, sleep, and concentration.Both anxiety and depression during menopause can be influenced by a history of mental health issues, lifestyle factors (such as stress and lack of physical activity), and psycho social factors, including stressful life events and cultural attitudes towards ageing and menopause.

Coping Strategies and Mental Health Support

Developing effective coping mechanisms can really help to maintain emotional well-being. Techniques may include stress management, (mindfulness, meditation and yoga) cognitive-behavioural therapy, and a balanced diet rich in omega-3 fatty acids. Social support from friends, family, or support groups can also provide a sense of community.

The role of mental health professionals in providing therapy and possibly medication is also worthy of consideration.

Yoga and Mindfulness for Menopause Relief

Yoga combines physical postures, breath control, and meditation to improve flexibility, strength, and balance while also reducing stress and anxiety. Mindfulness, the practice of being present and fully engaged with the current moment without judgment, can help manage menopausal symptoms by reducing stress and promoting a sense of calm and acceptance. I have also found journaling to be a useful habit to adopt.

Making changes is possible and adopting new habits can be powerful. Ultimately any change is up to you to choose. Try and plan some time just for you each day where you can focus on some of these suggestions.

Ten

Managing Vaginal Dryness and Painful Sex

In this chapter we talk about the intimate aspect of menopause—sexual health, addressing common concerns such as loss of interest in sex and painful sex, and offering solutions to these challenges to restore comfort and enjoyment to your relationships.

<u>Loss of interest in sex</u> : This can be a scary new experience but is a common issue during menopause, often resulting from hormonal changes. Lower levels of oestrogen and testosterone can reduce your interest in sex. Psychological factors like body image changes, stress, fatigue, and the emotional impact of other menopausal symptoms can also play a role. It is really important that you can speak openly with your partner and healthcare providers to find effective and comfortable solutions to help maintain a fulfilling sex life during and after menopause.

<u>**Painful Intercourse:**</u> Painful intercourse during menopause is frequently due to vaginal dryness and thinning of the vaginal walls, conditions collectively known as vaginal atrophy. Oestrogen helps maintain the thickness and lubrication of the vaginal lining, so when levels drop, these tissues can become less elastic, drier, and more susceptible to tearing or irritation. These changes can lead to discomfort or pain during sex, which can understandably diminish sexual desire and satisfaction.

Other Contributing Factors: Pain during sex may also be influenced by other menopausal symptoms, such as a decrease in sexual desire and emotional changes, which can affect arousal and the physical preparedness for sex. Additionally, certain medical conditions, like urinary tract infections or yeast infections, which may become more common during menopause, can also lead to painful sex.

Solutions for Sexual Issues During Menopause: There are many solutions to these problems. It can be a matter of trial and error to find the best solution for you and it may include combinations of the following:

- **Lubricants and Moisturizers:** The use of water-based lubricants during sex and regular application of vaginal moisturizers can alleviate dryness and discomfort. There are over-the-counter and prescription treatments which can help so speak with your healthcare professional about your options.
- **Topical Estrogen Therapy:** Applied directly to the vaginal tissues, this can help restore thickness and elasticity.
- **Systemic Hormone Replacement Therapy (HRT):** This

can address many symptoms of menopause, including those affecting sexual health, it should be considered thoughtfully with medical guidance.

- **Pelvic Floor Exercises:** Strengthening the pelvic floor muscles can improve sexual function and reduce discomfort.
- **Communication and Counselling**: Open communication with a partner about sexual needs and preferences, possibly facilitated by a counsellor or sex therapist, can be helpful.
- **Medical Interventions:** For some women, prescription medications designed to enhance interest in sex can be an option.

Eleven

Managing Bladder Symptoms

Bladder symptoms often become more prominent during menopause due to the decline in oestrogen levels, which can affect urinary tract health. The main bladder-related issues that can arise are increased frequency of urination, urinary incontinence, and urinary tract infections (UTIs).Bladder symptoms can be very distressing so it's important to seek advice from your healthcare practitioner if your quality of life is being affected.

Increased Frequency and Urgency: You may feel the need to pee more often, sometimes with an urgent sensation. This can be due to changes in the bladder and pelvic floor muscles.

Urinary Incontinence: There are several types of incontinence that can affect menopausal women:

- **Stress Incontinence:** Leaking urine during activities that put pressure on the bladder, like coughing, sneezing, laughing, or exercise.
- **Urge Incontinence:** A sudden, intense urge to pee followed by an involuntary loss of urine.
- **Mixed Incontinence:** A combination of stress and urge incontinence.

Urinary Tract Infections (UTI's) The changes in the vaginal flora and the thinning of the urethra can lead to an increased risk of UTIs. Symptoms of a UTI include a burning sensation when peeing, needing to pee frequently, and cloudy or strong-smelling pee.

Management Strategies

- Pelvic Floor Exercises: Kegel exercises can strengthen the pelvic floor muscles and reduce symptoms of stress incontinence.
- Bladder Training: This involves going to the bathroom at set times to train the bladder to control urges.
- Hydration: Drink plenty of fluids to stay hydrated but limit fluid intake in the evening if waking at night to pee is an issue.
- Diet: Avoid foods and drinks that can irritate the bladder, such as caffeine, alcohol, and acidic foods.
- Weight Management: Extra weight can increase pressure on the bladder and aggravate incontinence.
- Topical Oestrogen: For some women, using topical estrogen creams or rings can help improve the health of vaginal and urethral tissues.

- Medications: Certain medications can manage overactive bladder symptoms.
- Non-surgical Treatments: Vaginal pessaries or urethral inserts can help with incontinence.
- Surgical Options: In severe cases, surgery may be considered for stress incontinence.

Twelve

Menopausal Weight Gain

This chapter addresses the common issue of weight gain during menopause, exploring the underlying factors and providing strategies for managing weight through this transition. It provides information and practical tips for creating a balanced diet and exercise plan tailored to your individual needs. It will also discuss the psychological aspects of weight gain, offering you strategies to maintain a positive body image and set realistic weight management goals.

Menopausal Weight Gain: Weight gain during menopause is a frequent concern for many women and can be really stressful and tricky to navigate. Menopausal weight gain is a complex issue influenced by hormonal changes, ageing, and lifestyle factors. The decline in oestrogen levels is associated with a decrease in metabolic rate and an increase in abdominal fat. This central fat distribution is not only challenging to manage but is also associated with a higher risk for cardiovascular disease and diabetes.

Importance of Exercise: Regular physical activity is one of the most beneficial habits for managing menopausal symptoms. Exercise helps to regulate hormones, improve mood, enhance sleep quality, maintain a healthy weight, and promote cardio-vascular health. A combination of aerobic, strength-training, and flexibility exercises is recommended to cover all aspects of physical health.

The challenge in managing menopausal weight gain lies in finding the balance between sufficient exercise to counteract the metabolic slowdown without over-stressing the body. While cardiovascular exercise is essential for heart health and caloric burn, intense cardio can sometimes lead to increased cortisol levels, the stress hormone that can promote fat storage, particularly in the abdominal area.

To address this, it's important to shift the focus shifts from high-intensity workouts to low to moderate-intensity cardio exercises which are effective, yet less likely to cause undue stress on the body. Activities like brisk walking, cycling, swimming, or low-impact aerobics are great options. They elevate the heart rate and encourage fat burning without the potential negative impacts of high-intensity workouts, such as joint stress or excessive production of stress hormones.

In addition to aerobic activities, strength training is crucial as it builds muscle mass, which burns more calories than fat, even at rest. Weight-bearing exercises not only help with maintaining muscle mass but also contribute to bone density, which is particularly important to combat osteoporosis.

You should aim for a well-rounded fitness routine that includes moderate aerobic activity, strength training, flexibility exercises, and balance training. It's also essential to incorporate rest days to allow the body to recover and prevent over-training.

Metabolism Changes: As women age, their metabolic rate naturally slows down. This means that your body may require fewer calories for energy, making weight gain more likely if you keep eating the same way you always have. Menopause can further slow metabolism due to the loss of muscle mass that tends to occur with ageing.

Dietary Recommendations: Diet plays a crucial role in managing menopausal weight gain and overall health. As metabolism slows down during menopause, it becomes even more important to focus on diet quality, caloric intake, and nutritional balance.

As a disclaimer, I am not a nutrition expert, rather sharing my thoughts and experience from reading and trying things for myself. There are many experts with great subject matter to support healthy eating with recipes and meal plans, the reality is you have to choose to prioritise you and figure out what works for you as an individual.

A balanced diet rich in fruits, vegetables, whole grains, lean proteins, and healthy fats can be delicious and help manage weight. It's also important to limit processed foods, sugar, and saturated fats. You may find that smaller, more frequent meals help maintain energy levels and control your hunger. I have no desire to be the fun police when it comes to managing the food you eat and suggest that perhaps the 80:20 rule might be a good way to manage things. I've found it has been a great option for me. Make healthy food choices 80 percent of the time and indulge in whatever you deem to be a treat just 20 percent of the time. Making gradual, sustainable changes is the goal for long-term success.

Nutrient-Dense Foods: Your diet should prioritize nutrient-dense foods that provide vitamins, minerals, fibre, and other nutrients without too many calories. These include fruits, vegetables, lean proteins, whole grains, and healthy fats.

Protein Intake: Adequate protein can help maintain muscle mass, which is important as muscle burns more calories than fat. Good sources include lean meats, poultry, fish, beans, lentils, tofu, and low-fat dairy products. Protein supplements can also be helpful.

Complex Carbohydrates: Instead of simple sugars and refined carbs, choose complex carbohydrates like whole grains, legumes, and vegetables that provide lasting energy and fibre.

Healthy Fats: Incorporate sources of unsaturated fats, which are beneficial for heart health. These include nuts, seeds, avocados, olive oil, and fatty fish rich in omega-3 fatty acids.

Calcium and Vitamin D: These are essential for bone health, particularly during menopause. Sources of calcium include dairy products, fortified plant milks, leafy greens, and almonds. Vitamin D can be obtained from exposure to sunlight, fatty fish, and some fortified foods.

Limiting Alcohol and Sugar: Alcohol and sugary foods and beverages can contribute to weight gain and provide little nutritional value, so they should be consumed sparingly.

Strategies for Healthy Eating

- **Mindful Eating:** Pay attention to hunger and fullness cues to avoid overeating. Eat slowly and without distractions when possible.
- **Portion Control:** It's easy to consume more calories than needed when portions are large. Understanding and being mindful of portion sizes can help prevent overeating. Simple solutions to reducing portion sizes include using a smaller sized plate for your meals.
- **Hydration:** Drink plenty of water throughout the day. Sometimes thirst is mistaken for hunger, leading to overeating.
- **Meal Planning:** Plan your meals in advance to make healthier choices and prevent last-minute, less nutritious choices.
- **Meal Timing:** Eating regular meals and snacks can help maintain blood sugar levels and prevent overeating. You may find that eating a light dinner or eating earlier in the evening can help with weight management.
- **Cook at Home:** Preparing meals at home allows for control over ingredients and portion sizes.
- **Moderation:** It's important to enjoy all foods in moder-

ation, this helps to avoid feelings of deprivation that can derail healthy eating habits.

Thirteen

Managing Irregular Menstrual Cycles

Irregular menstrual cycles during the peri-menopausal phase—the years leading up to menopause—are a common experience for many women. This irregularity can affect changes in the duration of periods, the amount of blood flow, or the length of the cycle itself.

Understanding Irregular Menstrual Cycles:

- **Variations in Cycle Length:** You may notice that your periods come more closely together or are spaced further apart. Some cycles may be skipped altogether.
- **Changes in Flow:** Your periods may become lighter or heavier, and you might experience spotting between periods.
- **Hormonal Fluctuations:** These changes are typically due to fluctuations in oestrogen and progesterone levels as the

ovaries begin to reduce hormone production.

Management Strategies

- **Track Your Cycle:** Keeping a record can help identify patterns and help discussions with your healthcare provider.
- **Lifestyle Adjustments:** Regular exercise and maintaining a healthy weight can help regulate hormones and manage symptoms.
- **Stress Reduction:** Stress can exacerbate hormonal imbalances, so implementing stress-reduction techniques like yoga or meditation can be beneficial.
- **Diet:** Consuming a balanced diet rich in whole foods can support overall health and may help stabilize hormones.
- **Nonsteroidal Anti-inflammatory Drugs (NSAIDs):** These can help to reduce heavy menstrual bleeding and alleviate cramping, their use should be discussed with your healthcare provider.

Medical Interventions

- **Hormonal Contraceptives:** Birth control pills, patches, or rings can regulate menstrual cycles and help control heavy bleeding.: Taking progestin can help balance hormones and normalize menstrual cycles.
- **Endometrial Ablation:** In cases of heavy bleeding where you don't want to have any more children, this procedure can reduce menstrual flow or stop it entirely.
- **Hysterectomy:** In severe cases and when other treatments have failed, removal of the uterus may be considered to

resolve menstrual irregularities and associated symptoms.

It's important that you discuss irregular menstrual cycles with your healthcare provider to ensure that the changes are a normal part of menopause and not symptoms of other conditions.

Fourteen

Heart Health

In this chapter, we look at the crucial aspect of heart health during and after menopause, focusing on the increased risk of cardiovascular issues that accompany this life stage.

Increased Risk of Cardiovascular Issues: The decline in oestrogen during menopause is linked to an increased risk of cardiovascular disease (CVD). Oestrogen has a protective effect on the inner layer of artery walls, helping to keep blood vessels flexible. When levels fall, this can lead to changes in the walls of the blood vessels, making them more prone to atherosclerosis (hardening of the arteries).

Impact of Hormonal Changes on Heart Health: Hormonal changes during menopause can lead to an increase in blood pressure and changes in blood lipid levels, including increases in LDL ("bad" cholesterol) and decreases in HDL ("good" cholesterol). Each of these factors can contribute to the development of heart disease.

Risk of Heart Attack: Women are at an increased risk of heart attack after menopause. Oestrogen, which offers some protection against artery inflammation and keeps blood vessel walls flexible, decreases significantly during menopause. This can contribute to the build-up of plaque in the arteries, leading to atherosclerosis, which can eventually result in a heart attack.

Heart attacks in women can often go undiagnosed or be misdiagnosed. This is due to several factors:

- **Symptom Presentation:** Women may experience symptoms that are less commonly associated with heart attacks, such as nausea, shortness of breath, back or jaw pain, and fatigue, rather than the classic symptom of chest pain.
- **Under-Recognition:** Both women and healthcare providers may underestimate the risk of heart disease in women, leading to less aggressive pursuit of diagnosis and treatment compared to men.
- **Differences in Symptoms:** Women's heart attack symptoms can be subtler than men's and may be mistaken for less serious conditions, such as indigestion, anxiety, or menopausal changes.
- **Communication of Symptoms:** Women may describe their symptoms differently than men, and if they do not report classic chest pain, the possibility of a heart attack might not be immediately considered.
- **Lack of Awareness:** There is a general lack of public awareness that heart disease is as much of a health issue for

women as it is for men, which can contribute to delayed treatment. It's really important that you understand your cardiovascular risks post-menopause and are empowered to seek out advice for prevention.

Cardiovascular Disease Prevention: Prevention strategies include maintaining a healthy diet rich in fruits, vegetables, whole grains, lean proteins, and healthy fats; engaging in regular physical activity; quitting smoking; managing stress; and maintaining a healthy weight. Regular health screenings are also vital to monitor blood pressure, cholesterol levels, and other risk factors for heart disease.

Fifteen

Gynecological Health

This chapter covers the important changes occurring in your gynaecological health during menopause, changes to your reproductive system, the significance of postmenopausal bleeding, and the importance of continued screening for gynaecological cancers. It will also emphasize the importance of seeking prompt medical attention for any concerning symptoms and provide guidance on navigating healthcare decisions during this phase of your life.

Changes in the Reproductive System: Menopause signifies the end of your reproductive years, marked by the cessation of your periods. They can become irregular over a period of time as the hormonal changes lead to the ovaries no longer releasing eggs and producing less oestrogen and progesterone. These hormonal shifts can cause physical changes in the reproductive organs, such as the shrinking of the uterus and decreased elasticity of the vaginal tissues.

Uterine Changes: The uterus may decrease in size, and the endometrium (the lining of the uterus) no longer thickens each month, leading to the cessation of periods. Reduced hormone levels can also affect the uterine ligaments, potentially causing a shift in the position of the uterus.

Vaginal Changes: The vaginal walls become thinner, less elastic, and more fragile—a condition known as vaginal atrophy. This change can lead to dryness, inflammation, and discomfort, and it may increase the risk of vaginal infections due to alterations in pH levels and the vaginal flora.

Cervical Changes: The cervix undergoes changes as well, with the production of cervical mucus declining, which can impact the vaginal environment further.

Pelvic Floor Muscles: The muscles and tissues supporting the pelvic organs can weaken, sometimes leading to conditions such as urinary incontinence or pelvic organ prolapse. You may notice this if you sometimes pee when you cough or sneeze.

Postmenopausal Bleeding (PMB): Any bleeding that occurs at least 12 months after your periods have stopped due to menopause is considered abnormal and warrants medical evaluation. Postmenopausal bleeding can result from benign conditions such as atrophic vaginitis or uterine fibroids, but it can also be a symptom of more serious issues like endometrial hyperplasia or cancer.

Common causes of post-menopausal bleeding include:

- **Atrophic Vaginitis:** Thinning and inflammation of the vaginal walls due to decreased estrogen levels can lead to bleeding, especially after sexual intercourse.
- **Endometrial Atrophy:** As oestrogen levels decline, the lining of the uterus can become too thin, leading to bleeding.
- **Polyps:** These benign growths in the lining of the uterus or cervix can cause bleeding. They are common in post-menopausal women.
- **Endometrial Hyperplasia:** This is a thickening of the endometrium that can lead to bleeding. Some types of hyperplasia increase the risk of developing endometrial cancer.
- **Medication Side Effects:** Hormone therapies, including hormone replacement therapy (HRT) or tamoxifen, a drug used to treat breast cancer, can cause PMB.

Serious conditions associated with post-menopausal bleeding (PMB) include:

- **Endometrial Cancer:** PMB is a common symptom of endometrial cancer, especially in postmenopausal women.
- **Other Gynaecological Cancers:** While less common, PMB can also be a symptom of cervical or ovarian cancer.

<u>Gynaecological Cancers and Screenings:</u> The risk of certain types of gynaecological cancers, including ovarian and endometrial cancers, increases with age. Regular screenings, such as pelvic exams, Pap tests, and HPV tests, are essential for early detection. You should also be aware of the symptoms of gynaecological cancers, which can include pelvic pain, abnormal bleeding, and changes in bowel or bladder habits and should always seek advice from a healthcare professional if you begin experiencing any of these.

Sixteen

Alternative and Complementary Therapies

In this chapter we look at the role of alternative and complementary therapies in managing menopausal symptoms, offering a closer look at herbal remedies and acupuncture. Whilst there are many opportunities for choosing to try any one of these therapies independent of any help or advice, I would strongly recommend you work with a healthcare professional to help individualise a plan of care for your wellbeing that is personalised for you. Herbal remedies can interact with medications so may not be suitable for everyone and you may end up feeling worse rather than better.

Herbal Remedies: Herbal remedies have been used for centuries to allegedly alleviate various menopausal symptoms but there is little research that evidences their success. Natural health practitioners will be able to provide advice and support.

Some of the most commonly used herbs include:

- Black Cohosh
- Red Clover
- Dong Quai
- Evening Primrose
- Flaxseed
- Omega 3's
- Pollen extract

Soy: This is rich in isoflavones, which are phytoestrogens that may help balance hormone levels and reduce hot flashes.

Acupuncture: Acupuncture is a practice derived from traditional Chinese medicine that involves inserting thin needles into specific points on the body. It is theorized to work by stimulating the body's natural healing processes and altering neurotransmitter levels. Acupuncture may help to relieve symptoms such as:

- **Hot Flashes:** Some studies have found that acupuncture can reduce the frequency and severity of hot flashes.
- **Sleep Disturbances:** Acupuncture may improve sleep quality by reducing night sweats and calming the nervous system.
- **Mood Swings and Depression:** Acupuncture might help to regulate mood by affecting endorphin levels in the brain.

It is important to seek acupuncture treatment from qualified professionals and in conjunction with conventional medical advice.

Seventeen

Medical Interventions

In this chapter , we explore the medical interventions available to women experiencing menopausal symptoms, focusing on hormone replacement therapy (HRT), non-hormonal medications, and surgical options. Any of these treatments will require medical oversight and support and should be based on your individual health status, risk factors, severity of your symptoms, your personal preferences, and the balance of your individual risks and benefits.

Hormone Replacement Therapy (HRT): HRT involves the administration of estrogen and, often, progesterone to alleviate menopausal symptoms. It is one of the most effective treatments for managing hot flashes, night sweats, and vaginal symptoms and is well tolerated by many women. HRT can be systemic (pills, patches, gels, sprays) or local (vaginal creams, tablets, or rings). However, HRT is not suitable for everyone, and its use must be carefully considered against potential risks, such as an increased risk of breast cancer, blood clots, and stroke, particularly with long-term use.

Non-hormonal Medications for Symptom Relief: For women who cannot or prefer not to use HRT, there are non-hormonal medications that can help alleviate certain menopausal symptoms:

- **Antidepressants:** Certain low-dose antidepressants may reduce hot flashes and are helpful for mood swings or depression.
- **Gabapentin:** Originally used for seizure disorders, it can be effective for hot flashes and night sweats.
- **Clonidine:** Typically used to treat high blood pressure, it can also provide relief for some women with hot flashes.

The availability of these medications will be governed by the country you live in so you should speak with your doctor if you want to pursue some of these options.

Surgical Options: In certain cases, surgical interventions may be necessary or chosen for various gynaecological reasons:

- **Hysterectomy:** Removal of the uterus. This surgery is undertaken for various reasons, such as fibroids, heavy bleeding or cancer, but it does not induce menopause unless the ovaries are also removed.
- **Oophorectomy:** Removal of the ovaries, which does induce menopause. This surgery may be performed due to the risk of or presence of ovarian cancer or other significant

pelvic problems.

Eighteen

Preventive Healthcare for Post-Menopausal Women

In this chapter we will cover information on each recommended screening and aspect of preventive care, providing guidance on how frequently these should be undertaken. It will also underscore the critical role that lifestyle choices play in preventive health and the importance of maintaining a dialogue with healthcare providers about what screenings and preventive measures are appropriate for individual health needs and concerns.

Screening Recommendations for post-menopausal women: As women enter the postmenopausal phase, they are advised to undergo regular health screenings that include:

- **Mammograms:** To screen for breast cancer, typically recommended every one to two years starting at age 50, or earlier for those with a family history or other risk factors.

- **Bone Density Scans (DEXA):** To assess bone health and the risk of osteoporosis, especially for women over the age of 65 or younger women with risk factors.
- **Colonoscopies:** To screen for colorectal cancer, starting at age 50, or earlier if there is a family history or other risk factors.
- **Cervical Cancer Screening:** Though less frequent for postmenopausal women, Pap smears should continue until at least the age of 65, depending on previous screening results and risk factors.
- **Blood Pressure Checks:** To monitor for hypertension, which becomes more common and carries greater risks as women age.
- **Lipid Profiles:** To screen for high cholesterol levels, which are a risk factor for cardiovascular disease.
- **Diabetes Screening:** Blood glucose tests are important, as the risk of type 2 diabetes increases with age.

Preventive Care for Aging Women: Preventive care extends beyond screenings to include:

- **Vaccinations:** Such as the flu vaccine, tetanus-diphtheria, pneumococcal vaccine, and shingles vaccine, according to age and medical guidelines and depending on your view of vaccinations.
- **Lifestyle Modifications:** Including a balanced diet, regular physical activity, smoking cessation, and moderate alcohol consumption, to prevent chronic diseases.
- **Mental Health:** Regular assessments for depression and anxiety are vital, as mental health is as important as physical

health.

- **Eye and Dental Exams:** Regular check-ups can prevent common age-related problems like glaucoma, cataracts, dry eye and gum disease.

Throughout this journey through menopause and beyond, it's important to have a positive trusted relationship with your healthcare provider so that you can seek the advice, support and treatment you need to navigate your way through this challenging stage of life and live well.

Nineteen

Conclusion

Thank you for reading this book. I genuinely hope you have found it helpful and that you are encouraged to explore options for yourself with more confidence.

If you have learned one thing you didn't know, please tell a friend, they too might not know about it.

The only way we can improve women's experiences and care during menopause and beyond, is by finding our collective voices and advocating for better education and acknowledgement of the significance of this important part of a woman's life.

If you have found this book useful I'd be very appreciative if you left a favourable review on Amazon.

Twenty

Resources

❧

Andy-Jb. (2015, November 25). *Treating hot flushes without hormones: What works, what doesn't.* British Menopause Society. https://thebms.org.uk/2015/09/treating-hot-flushes-without-hormones-what-works-what-doesnt/

Bda. (n.d.). *Menopause and diet.* https://www.bda.uk.com/resource/menopause-diet.html

Clear, J. (2018a). *Atomic Habbits.* Penguin Random House.

Let's Talk Mammograms. (2023, October 24). [Video]. https://www.hopkinsmedicine.org/health/treatment-tests-and-therapies/mammogram-procedure

Mariette-Jb. (2023, November 3). *British Menopause Society | For healthcare professionals and others specialising in post reproductive health.* British Menopause Society. https://thebms.org.uk/

Menopause and Eye Health | The North American Menopause Society, NAMS. (n.d.). https://www.menopause.org/for-wo men/menopauseflashes/women's-health-and-menopau se/menopause-and-eye-health

North American Menopause Society (NAMS) - Focused on Providing Physicians, Practitioners & Women Menopause Information, Help & Treatment Insights. (n.d.). https://www.menopause.org/

OpenAI. (2023). *ChatGPT* (November 14)[Large language model]. https://chat.openai.com

Professional, C. C. M. (n.d.-a). *Colonoscopy.* Cleveland Clinic. https://my.clevelandclinic.org/health/diagnostics/4949-colon oscopy

Professional, C. C. M. (n.d.-b). *Colonoscopy.* Cleveland Clinic. https://my.clevelandclinic.org/health/diagnostics/4949-colon oscopy

About the Author

Deborah Boyd is a RN who is passionate about women's health and advocating for women to have control over their well-being choices.

www.ingramcontent.com/pod-product-compliance
Lightning Source LLC
Chambersburg PA
CBHW050849260726
48660CB00006B/2526